50 Everyday Paleo Panini Recipes

Easy and Delicious Meals Everyone will Love

Disclaimer

Summary

Healthy eating and healthy living play a big role in the Paleo way of life and you'll find that opting for the Paleo diet is a big step towards eating the kinds of food items that was meant for your body to subside on in more primitive years.

However, you don't have to stick to salads and shakes and juices to get the right amount of nutrients, you can also enjoy delicious sandwiches, burgers and other food items.

Panini, in particular, is a kind of Italian sandwich which is becoming an exceedingly popular component of Paleo diets. Considered to be an extremely flexible and easy to make, whether you're looking for a quick snack, a refreshing and light lunch or just a lovely dinner, you can find recipes for Panini's almost everywhere.

With the help of this eBook, we'll acquaint you with the delicious world of Panini's and how you can incorporate them into your Paleo diet.

Table of Contents

50 Everyday Paleo Panini Recipes 1

Easy and Delicious Meals Everyone will Love.. 1

Summary 3

Understanding the Paleo Diet 7

Paleo Panini's 7

Making Paleo Panini Bread At Home 9

Avocado and Spinach Panini 11

Apple, Brie and Bacon Omelette Panini 13

Caprese Panini 15

Mozzarella, Shrimp and Avocado Panini...17

Turkey, Bacon and Chipotle Panini 19

Chicken Pesto Panini..21

Chicken and Rosemary Panini with Spinach and Sun Dried Tomatoes...............23

Turkey Panini with Citrus Aioli and Water Cress 24

Mediterranean Tuna Panini...27

Open Faced Panini with Turkey, Roasted Peppers, Spicy olives and Goat Cheese Topping 29

Prosciutto and Smoked Gouda Panini...31

Chicken Panini with Fig Jam 33

Manchego and Mushroom Panini..35

Spinach and Roast Chicken Panini 37

Roast Beef Panini 39

Basil and Pepper Panini...41

Basil Pesto and Portobello Mushroom Panini...43

Beani Panini...45

Classic Reuben Panini...47

Buffalo Chicken Panini...49

Grilled Asparagus and Prosciutto Panini...51

Ham and Brie Panini...53

Vegan Panini with an Olive Tapenade Spread and Caramelized Onions...55

Braised Short Rib Panini...57

Green Chile Steak Melt Panini...59

Prosciutto Wrapped Turkey and Avocado Panini...61

Red Chile Chicken Panini...63

Spinach and Chicken Panini with Lemon Herbs...66

Barbecued Salmon Panini...67

Crispy Fish Panini...70

Mango and Avocado Panini with Grilled Crabs...71

Heirloom Tomato Panini...73

Avocado and Mashed Chickpea Panini...75

BBQ Chicken Panini...78

Italian Grilled Pork Panini...81

Egg and Salmon Panini...82

BLT (Bacon, Lettuce and Tomato) Panini...84

Mediterranean Melt Panini...85

Muffeletta Panini...87

Pickled Onion Salad with Patty Melt Panini...89

Grilled Vegetable Panini...90

Caesar Shrimp and Arugula Panini 92

Salmon Salad Panini..95

Salmon BLT Panini 96

Green Goddess Grilled Cheese Panini 98

Tomato, Feta and Oregano Panini 100

Simple Salami Panini 103

Horse radish, Roast beef and Cheddar Panini 104

Understanding the Paleo Diet

The Paleo Diet is not a very complicated diet to understand. It's main aim and purpose is to help us connect to our earlier, primitive and wilder roots and to re-learn to exist on the diet that our ancestors subsided on.

Without tools and much technology, grains were almost non-existent. On the other hand, vegetables, fruits, meats and other food items that are attained through natural means make a large part of one's diet.

Processed food items such as cheese, ice-cream, yogurt, chocolate and other similar items aren't included in the diet since our ancestors would probably not have had these food items in their diets. Another thing that you should understand is that Paleo is not just a simple diet. Paleo is a whole other way of living.

Other than maintaining a very strict diet, Paleo also incorporates active exercises in the daily routine as well. This also holds on to the belief that our ancestors were predatory beings and living in a world where the rules of *"hunt or be hunted'* greatly applied.

However, nowadays, with no such danger threatening our existence, Paleo exercises are designed to mimic the strenuous activities of our forefathers. To truly benefit from the Paleo diet, it's always advisable to go the whole mile and do Paleo exercises as well.

Paleo Panini's

Many people think that Paleo diets must be rather bland. However, that's far from the truth. Paleo diets are known for incorporating food items that give you all the nutrients that your body needs and more. Another plus point is that you can still continue to eat burgers, pastas and other dishes as well, as long as you use the ingredients that are mentioned in your Paleo diet.

If you're a fan of sandwiches, then you obviously must be feeling pretty detached from your favorite food item. Sandwiches are extremely versatile, easy to make and can be eaten for breakfast, lunch dinner or just as a snack too. Paleo Panini's happen to be the most favored sandwiches in the Paleo diet. Furthermore, Panini's are made from bread that does not have grains and since the Paleo diet requires you to cut out all grains, this really comes as a welcome food item. Their ease of use and the many variations that you can try with the Panini to make a new sandwich make it a general favorite among every one.

If you're looking for great Panini recipes for your Paleo diet or even great Panini's to have on a daily basis then you'll definitely love the recipes that we've got in this eBook for you.

Making Paleo Panini Bread At Home

When you're looking to incorporate Paninis into your Paleo diet, you might have a bit of a challenge trying to find the proper Panini bread. Since the Paleo diet is very restrictive against most processed food items, it's not always possible to just rummage the fridge or head on down to the nearest store for bread. While it is possible to buy special Paleo bread in the market, you can also use the following recipe and make your own Paleo bread to use for Paninis or any other sandwich.

Nutritional Value per Serving:

Calories: 159

Carbohydrates: 12.0g,

Fat: 13.2g

Saturated Fat: 2.1g

Sodium: 113.2mg

Protein: 3.1g

Fiber: 7.7g

Sugar: 2.6g

Serving Size: 1 loaf

Preparation Time: 10 minutes

Cooking Time: 40 minutes

Ingredients

Almond flour	2 cups
Coconut flour	3 tablespoons
Ground flaxmeal	¼ cup

Sea salt	¼ teaspoon
Baking Soda	½ teaspoon
Organic eggs	5
Coconut oil	1 tablespoon
Raw honey	2 tablespoons
Apple cider vinegar	1 tablespoon

Method:

Grease up a baking pan or a loaf pan measuring 7.5x3.5 inches. Add the almond flour, ground flaxmeal, coconut flour, baking soda and the sea salt and mix them together in a food processor. Add in the eggs, the raw honey, coconut oil and the apple cider vinegar. Mix the ingredients well until you get a nice smooth batter.

Scoop out all the batter and put it in the greased loaf pan you prepared. Pop it in the oven at 350F for 30-35 minutes or until it's baked completely through. Let the bread rest on a bread rack to cool a bit before you use it.

You can also store it in an air-tight container for a few days.

Avocado and Spinach Panini

Nutritional Value per Serving:

Calories: 177,

Carbohydrates: 12.0g,

Fat: 14.9g

Saturated Fat: 2.1g

Sodium: 113.2mg

Protein: 3.1g

Fiber: 7.7g

Sugar: 2.6g

Serving Size: 4

Preparation Time: 15 minutes

Cooking Time: 25 minutes

Ingredients

Avocados	2 (thinly sliced and halved)
Sun-dried tomatoes	1/3 cup
Red Onions	2 tablespoons (diced)
Baby Spinach	2 cups (lightly packed)
Ciabatta rolls	16 ounce (split in half)
Salt and Pepper	According to taste

Method:

Spray the Panini bread with some cooking spray and then layer it with onions, avocados and ½ cup of the spinach. If you have a Panini maker, then just put the sandwich in it and cook for 4 minutes.

If you don't have a Panini maker, take a grilling pan or a skillet and coat it well with cooking spray. Let it come up to medium heat then place the Panini inside it. Take a smaller saucepan and place it on top of the Panini to compress it.

Make sure to weigh the smaller saucepan down to really compress the sandwich. Cook for 3-4minutes and then remove weight and cook the other side for 2-3 minutes, using the same technique.

Serve:

Serve hot or cold with a small spinach, dried tomatoes and onion salad made from any leftover ingredients.

Apple, Brie and Bacon Omelette Panini

Nutritional Value per Serving:

Calories: 710,

Carbohydrates: 42g

Cholesterol: 522mg

Fat: 44g

Saturated Fat: 22g

Sodium: 1510mg

Protein: 36g

Fiber: 3g

Serving Size: 2

Preparation Time: 15 minutes

Cooking Time: 30-35 minutes

Ingredients

Bacon strips	6
Butter	1 teaspoon
Eggs	4 (beaten)
Baby Spinach	2 cups (lightly packed)
Sourdough bread	4 slices (3/4 inches thick)
Brie	3 slices (Sliced thinly)
Apple	8 slices (sliced thinly)
Fresh baby spinach	½ cup

Softened butter	2 tablespoons
Salt and Pepper	According to taste

Method:

Over medium heat, cook the bacon first in a large skillet until it becomes crisp. Set aside to rest on paper towels to drain their oil.

Now take the skillet and heat up some butter on it still keeping it at a medium heat. Once the butter melts, pour in the eggs and stir slowly until the eggs start to cook.

Take the eggs off the heat once they're done and put them on two slices of the sour dough bread. Layer the remaining ingredients (apple, spinach, bri cheese) and use the remaining butter to grease the sandwich on the top and bottom.

If you have a Panini maker, cook on it until you see the cheese starting to melt and the bread turning brown.

If you don't have a Panini maker, take a grilling pan or a skillet and coat it well with cooking spray. Let it come up to medium heat then place the Panini inside it. Take a smaller saucepan and place it on top of the Panini to compress it.

Make sure to weigh the smaller saucepan down to really compress the sandwich. Cook for 3-4minutes and then remove weight and cook the other side for 2-3 minutes, using the same technique.

Serve:

Serve hot or cold with a small spinach, apples and brie salad made from any leftover ingredients.

Caprese Panini

Nutritional Value per Serving:

Calories: 582,

Carbohydrates: 33g

Cholesterol: 57mg

Fat: 37g

Saturated Fat: 12g

Sodium: 972mg

Protein: 29g

Fiber: 3g

Serving Size: 2

Preparation Time: 15 minutes

Cooking Time: 25 minutes

Ingredients

Balsamic vinegar	½ cup
Butter	1 teaspoon
Fresh basil leaves	6-8 (large)
Fresh Mozzarella	4 slices (3/4 inches thick)
Tomato	1 (large and sliced thinly)
Baguette	4 slices
Olive oil	2 tablespoons (for brushing only)
Salt and Pepper	According to taste

Method:

To reduce the balsamic vinegar, take a small saucepan and heat up the vinegar. Let it come up to a simmer and simmer it for 4 minutes or until it thickens. Keep an eye on the vinegar since it can burn easily. Take off heat and set aside once it has reduced to down to almost 4 tablespoons.

Take the Panini bread and drizzle some balsamic vinegar and olive oil inside before you start placing the basil leaves, tomatoes and mozzarella. Once it's ready, brush the Panini, with the olive oil on both sides.

If you have a Panini maker, cook on it until you see the cheese starting to melt and the bread turning brown.

If you don't have a Panini maker, take a grilling pan or a skillet and coat it well with cooking spray. Let it come up to medium heat then place the Panini inside it. Take a smaller saucepan and place it on top of the Panini to compress it.

Make sure to weigh the smaller saucepan down to really compress the sandwich. Cook for 3-4minutes and then remove weight and cook the other side for 2-3 minutes, using the same technique.

Serve:

Serve hot or cold with a small basil and goat cheese salad made from any leftover ingredients.

Mozzarella, Shrimp and Avocado Panini

Nutritional Value per Serving:

Calories: 400,

Carbohydrates: 36g

Cholesterol: 30mg

Fat: 26g

Saturated Fat: 8g

Sodium: 230mg

Protein: 11g

Fiber: 8g

Serving Size: 2

Preparation Time: 15 minutes

Cooking Time: 45 minutes

Ingredients

Ripe avocados	2-3 (pitted, peeled and mashed)
Roma tomato	1 (deseeded and diced)
Fresh lemon juice	1½ tablespoon
Minced garlic	½ teaspoon
Mozzarella	6 slices
Sour dough bread	4 or 6 slices
Olive oil	2 tablespoons (for brushing only)
Extra large shrimps	6 (cooked and halved, lengthwise)

Salt and Pepper	According to taste
Red pepper flakes	According to taste

Method:

Combine the mashed avocado, the garlic and teaspoon of the lemon juice together in a small bowl. Season it with salt, red pepper flakes and pepper according to your taste and set aside. Take the cooked shrimps and drizzle the remaining lemon juice on them. Toss them well to make sure that they are all coated with it.

Take two slices of bread and brush them with oil on both sides. Place a slice of mozzarella cheese on the bread and then spoon some of the avocado mixture on to the cheese. Add another slice of mozzarella and then layer with the shrimp. Add the third slice of cheese and top off with a slice of bread.

If you have a Panini maker, cook on it until you see the cheese starting to melt and the bread turning brown.

If you don't have a Panini maker, take a grilling pan or a skillet and coat it well with cooking spray. Let it come up to medium heat then place the Panini inside it. Take a smaller saucepan and place it on top of the Panini to compress it.

Make sure to weigh the smaller saucepan down to really compress the sandwich. Cook for 3-4minutes and then remove weight and cook the other side for 2-3 minutes, using the same technique.

Serve:

Serve hot or cold with a cold glass of lemonade and guacamole or some other avocado dip.

Turkey, Bacon and Chipotle Panini

Nutritional Value per Serving:

Calories: 601,

Carbohydrates: 62.7g

Cholesterol: 70mg

Fat: 23.2g

Saturated Fat: 0g

Sodium: 2074mg

Protein: 34.2g

Fiber: 4.1g

Serving Size: 4

Preparation Time: 15 minutes

Cooking Time: 25 minutes

Ingredients

Bacon	8 slices
Butter	1 tablespoon
Red Onion	½ cup (thinly sliced)
Garlic	2 cloves (minced)
Fresh spinach leaves	3 cups
Mayonnaise	½ cup (reduced fat)
Olive oil	2 tablespoons (for brushing only)
Chipotle peppers	2 (minced and in adobo sauce)

Adobo sauce	1 teaspoon (use the one that you soaked the peppers in)
Focaccia bread	8 slices
Provolone cheese	4 slices
Turkey	½ pound (sliced, deli meat)
Salt and Pepper	According to taste
Red pepper flakes	According to taste

Method:

Cook off the bacon on medium heat in a normal sized saucepan until it turns nice and brown. Set the bacon aside on paper towels. Take a skillet and melt some butter in it. Add the onions and garlic and keep cooking for 10 minutes or until the onions begin to turn translucent. Add the spinach leaves now and keep cooking for another 3 minutes or until the leaves begin to wilt a bit.

Take the bacon and divide it so that one sandwich gets two strips of bacon. Now take the adobo sauce, the chipotle peppers and the mayonnaise and mix them well together in a bowl. Take the mayonnaise and spread it on the bread slices. Place a slice of cheese on the bread and a portion of the turkey deli meat. Put two strips of bacon and spoon some of the spinach mixture on top. Place the bread slice on top and oil both sides of the sandwich.

If you have a Panini maker, cook on it until you see the cheese starting to melt and the bread turning brown. If you don't have a Panini maker, take a grilling pan or a skillet and coat it well with cooking spray. Let it come up to medium heat then place the Panini inside it. Take a smaller saucepan and place it on top of the Panini to compress it.

Make sure to weigh the smaller saucepan down to really compress the sandwich. Cook for 3-4minutes and then remove weight and cook the other side for 2-3 minutes, using the same technique.

Serve:

Serve hot or cold with your favorite beverage.

Chicken Pesto Panini

Nutritional Value per Serving:

Calories: 641,

Carbohydrates: 60.9g

Cholesterol: 61mg

Fat: 29.4g

Saturated Fat: 0g

Sodium: 1076mg

Protein: 32.4g

Fiber: 4.4g

Serving Size: 4

Preparation Time: 10 minutes

Cooking Time: 25 minutes

Ingredients

Chicken	1 cup (cooked and diced)
Basil pesto	½ cup (pre-prepared solution)
Green bell pepper	½ cup (diced)
Red Onion	¼ cup (diced)
Monterey Jack cheese	1 cup (shredded)
Olive oil	2 tablespoons (for brushing only)
Focaccia bread	8 slices

Salt and Pepper   According to taste

Method:

Take the bread for the sandwich and layer the bottom half with pesto, chicken, onion, green bell pepper and sprinkle some shredded cheese on top of it. Make sure you layer them in an equal amount. Now add the top half of the bread. Use the olive oil to lightly grease the bread sides.

If you have a Panini maker, cook on it until you see the cheese starting to melt and the bread turning brown. If you don't have a Panini maker, take a grilling pan or a skillet and coat it well with cooking spray. Let it come up to medium heat then place the Panini inside it. Take a smaller saucepan and place it on top of the Panini to compress it.

Make sure to weigh the smaller saucepan down to really compress the sandwich. Cook for 3-4minutes and then remove weight and cook the other side for 2-3 minutes, using the same technique.

Serve:

Serve hot or cold with your favorite beverage.

Chicken and Rosemary Panini with Spinach and Sun Dried Tomatoes

Nutritional Value per Serving:

Calories: 414,

Carbohydrates: 33.6g

Cholesterol: 77mg

Fat: 14.8g

Saturated Fat: 3.9g

Sodium: 687mg

Protein: 32.4g

Fiber: 3.1g

Preparation Time: 15 minutes

Cooking Time: 25 minutes

Ingredients

Chicken cutlets	4 (cooked and diced)
Sun dried tomato	¼ cup (oil packed, drained, chopped)
Fresh rosemary	½ cup (diced)
Red pepper	1/8 teaspoon (crushed)
Garlic cloves	8 (thinly sliced)
Extra virgin olive oil	2 tablespoons (for brushing only)
Fresh baby spinach	1 packet (6 oz)
Salt and Pepper	According to taste
Italian bread	8 slices

Mozzarella cheese	½ cup (shredded)

Method:

Take a zip lock bag and combine the chicken, rosemary and 2 teaspoons of olive oil. Seal the bag and set it aside to marinate for 30 minutes in the fridge.

Take the remaining olive oil and heat it up in a skillet. Heat the skillet to medium-high and sauté the red pepper, garlic and sun-dried tomatoes for 5 minutes or until the garlic turns brown. Season the mixture with salt and pepper before taking it off the heat and setting it aside.

In the same pan, add some more oil or use a cooking spray to grease it. Take out the chicken and cook it for 3 minutes on each side or until golden brown in color. Season with salt and pepper and set aside.

Take some bread and start layering it to make your Panini. Add one tablespoon of shredded cheese, one cutlet of chicken, spoon on some sun-dried tomato mixture and add the top half of the bread.

If you have a Panini maker, cook on it until you see the cheese starting to melt and the bread turning brown. If you don't have a Panini maker, take a grilling pan or a skillet and coat it well with cooking spray. Let it come up to medium heat then place the Panini inside it. Take a smaller saucepan and place it on top of the Panini to compress it.

Make sure to weigh the smaller saucepan down to really compress the sandwich. Cook for 3-4minutes and then remove weight and cook the other side for 2-3 minutes, using the same technique.

Serve:

Serve hot or cold with your favorite beverage.

Turkey Panini with Citrus Aioli and Water Cress
Nutritional Value per Serving:

Calories: 304,

Carbohydrates: 33.6g

Cholesterol: 38mg

Fat: 11.8g

Saturated Fat: 2.7g

Sodium: 810mg

Protein: 21.3g

Fiber: 1.2g

Serving Size: 4

Preparation Time: 15 minutes

Cooking Time: 25 minutes

Ingredients

Lemon rind	¼ teaspoon (grated)
Lime rind	¼ teaspoon (grated)
Canola mayonnaise	2 tablespoons
Fresh lemon juice	1 teaspoon
Watercress	2 cups (trimmed)
Garlic cloves	1
Extra virgin olive oil	2 tablespoons (for brushing only)
Turkey	½ pound (sliced, deli meat)
Provolone cheese	4 slices

Salt and Pepper	According to taste
Italian bread	8 slices

Method:

Take a small bowl and combine the lemon rind, the lime rind, the canola mayonnaise, some black pepper, and the lemon juice and mix them well together. Once they're thoroughly mixed, set them aside.

Take some bread and start layering it to make your Panini. Add the shredded cheese, water cress and turkey and add the top half of the bread.

If you have a Panini maker, cook on it until you see the cheese starting to melt and the bread turning brown. If you don't have a Panini maker, take a grilling pan or a skillet and coat it well with cooking spray. Let it come up to medium heat then place the Panini inside it. Take a smaller saucepan and place it on top of the Panini to compress it.

Make sure to weigh the smaller saucepan down to really compress the sandwich. Cook for 3-4minutes and then remove weight and cook the other side for 2-3 minutes, using the same technique.

Serve:

Serve hot or cold with your favorite beverage.

Mediterranean Tuna Panini

Nutritional Value per Serving:

Calories: 336,

Carbohydrates: 35g

Cholesterol: 61mg

Fat: 6g

Saturated Fat: 2g

Sodium: 543mg

Protein: 34g

Fiber: 5g

Serving Size: 4

Preparation Time: 10 minutes

Cooking Time: 25 minutes

Ingredients

Tuna	2 cans (6 oz each, light, drained)
Plum tomato	1 (chopped)
Feta cheese	¼ cup (crumbled)
Fresh lemon juice	1 teaspoon
Artichoke hearts	2 tablespoons (chopped, marinated)
Red Onion	2 tablespoons (minced)
Kalamata olives	1 tablespoon (pitted and chopped)
Capers	1 teaspoon (chopped and rinsed)

Canola oil	2 tablespoons
Salt and Pepper	According to taste
Italian bread	8 slices

Method:

Start off by flaking the tuna with the help of a fork. Once all the tuna has been flaked, add in the olives, onions, capers, artichokes, feta, lemon juice and some salt pepper. Mix them well until all the ingredients are combined. Take some bread and spread some of the tuna mixture on it. Add the top layer and set aside to cook.

If you have a Panini maker, cook on it until you see the cheese starting to melt and the bread turning brown. If you don't have a Panini maker, take a grilling pan or a skillet and coat it well with cooking spray. Let it come up to medium heat then place the Panini inside it. Take a smaller saucepan and place it on top of the Panini to compress it.

Make sure to weigh the smaller saucepan down to really compress the sandwich. Cook for 3-4minutes and then remove weight and cook the other side for 2-3 minutes, using the same technique.

Serve:

Serve hot or cold with your favorite beverage.

Open Faced Panini with Turkey, Roasted Peppers, Spicy olives and Goat Cheese Topping

Nutritional Value per Serving:

Calories: 126,

Carbohydrates: 18.1g

Cholesterol: 4mg

Fat: 4.4g

Saturated Fat: 2g

Sodium: 420mg

Protein: 4g

Fiber: 1.8g

Serving Size: 4

Preparation Time: 20 minutes

Cooking Time: 25 minutes

Ingredients

Red bell peppers	2 (de-seeded and chopped in to half, lengthwise only)
Olives	6 (minced, pitted, ripe)
Green olives	8 (minced, pitted)
Fresh lemon juice	2 teaspoons
Fresh basil	1 tablespoon (minced)
Lemon rind	2 teaspoons
Red pepper	1/8 teaspoon (ground)

Garlic	1 (small, minced)
Goat's cheese	3 tablespoons (crumbled)
Salt and Pepper	According to taste
Italian bread	8 slices

Method:

Take the bell peppers and place them, skin side up on a baking sheet lined with foil. Broil the bell peppers for 15 minutes or until they start to blacken a bit. Take them out and place them in a zip lock bag. Set aside for 10 minutes before peeling them and cutting them into strips. Mix some salt with the chopped peppers and set aside.

Combine the ripe olives, the garlic, green olives, the lemon rind, fresh basil and the fresh lemon juice in a small bowl.

If you have a Panini maker, only cook the bread on it until it turns brown. If you don't have a Panini maker, take a grilling pan or a skillet and coat it well with cooking spray. Let it come up to medium heat then place the Panini inside it.

However, since we're making an open faced Panini sandwich, we won't need to add a top layer or apply pressure since you'll only need bread for one side of the sandwich.

Once the bread turns golden, take it out and place one spoonful of the olive mixture and top off with the salted pepper strips and some goat's cheese on top.

Serve:

Serve hot or cold with your favorite beverage.

Prosciutto and Smoked Gouda Panini

Nutritional Value per Serving:

Calories: 265

Carbohydrates: 28.9g

Cholesterol: 36mg

Fat: 9.7g

Saturated Fat: 5g

Sodium: 722mg

Protein: 14.5g

Fiber: 1.5g

Serving Size: 4

Preparation Time: 15 minutes

Cooking Time: 15 minutes

Ingredients

Smoked, Gouda cheese	6 slices
Prosciutto	6 slices (extremely thin)
Olive oil	2 tablespoons
Salt and Pepper	According to taste
Italian bread	8 slices

Method:

There's not much preparation involved with this and you can easily take the prosciutto and the Gouda and layer their slices according to the kind of texture you're looking for.

One slice of Gouda and two prosciutto slices would make the Panini meatier in taste and texture. On the other hand, prosciutto with two slices of Gouda cheese would get more of the smoky cheesy texture of the Gouda cheese. Once you're happy with the layering, brush both sides of the sandwich with olive oil.

If you have a Panini maker, cook on it until you see the cheese starting to melt and the bread turning brown.

If you don't have a Panini maker, take a grilling pan or a skillet and coat it well with cooking spray. Let it come up to medium heat then place the Panini inside it. Take a smaller saucepan and place it on top of the Panini to compress it.

Make sure to weigh the smaller saucepan down to really compress the sandwich. Cook for 3-4minutes and then remove weight and cook the other side for 2-3 minutes, using the same technique.

Serve:

Serve hot or cold with your favorite beverage.

Chicken Panini with Fig Jam

Nutritional Value per Serving:

Calories: 381,

Carbohydrates: 42.6g

Cholesterol: 70mg

Fat: 12.7g

Saturated Fat: 6.1g

Sodium: 591mg

Protein: 24.7g

Fiber: 1.2g

Serving Size: 4

Preparation Time: 15 minutes

Cooking Time: 25 minutes

Ingredients

Fig jam	¼ cup slices
Butter	2 tablespoons (softened)
Blue cheese	¼ cup (crumbled)
Chicken breast	8 oz. (cooked, chopped)
Lemon juice	1 teaspoon
Arugula leaves	2 cups
Olive oil	2 tablespoons
Salt and Pepper	According to taste

Ciabatta bread   8 slices

Method:

Spread the jam on the bread, making sure to apply it on the top halves only. Take a small bowl and combined the softened butter and the cheese. Stir thoroughly until you get a smooth mixture.

Spread this cheese mixture on the bottom half of the bread only. Take the chopped chicken breasts and arrange them as evenly as possible over the cheese spread layer. Season the chicken meat with some salt and pepper. Add on the top layer with the fig jam on it and oil both sides with some olive oil

If you have a Panini maker, cook on it until you see the bread turning brown. If you don't have a Panini maker, take a grilling pan or a skillet and coat it well with cooking spray. Let it come up to medium heat then place the Panini inside it. Take a smaller saucepan and place it on top of the Panini to compress it.

Make sure to weigh the smaller saucepan down to really compress the sandwich. Cook for 3-4minutes and then remove weight and cook the other side for 2-3 minutes, using the same technique.

Serve:

Serve hot or cold with your favorite beverage.

Manchego and Mushroom Panini

Nutritional Value per Serving:

Calories: 352

Carbohydrates: 48.8g

Cholesterol: 25mg

Fat: 10.9g

Saturated Fat: 6g

Sodium: 741mg

Protein: 16.8g

Fiber: 3.7g

Serving Size: 4

Preparation Time: 10minutes

Cooking Time: 20minutes

Ingredients:

Mushroom blend	4 ounce package (could be oyster, shiitake and cremini)
Manchego cheese	3 ounces
Cremini musrooms	8 ounce (presliced package)
Vinegar	1 ½ tbsp
Fresh garlic	2 tbsp (minced)
Fresh thyme	1 tbsp (chopped)
Sea salt and pepper	According to taste
Butter	1 tbsp

Shallots	¼ cup (minced)
Sourdough bread	8 slices

Method:

Heat up butter and add shallots, salt, pepper, thyme, mushrooms, mushroom blend and garlic. Cook for about 10 minutes and till the water disappears. Then add vinegar and cook for 30 more seconds.

Pour mushroom mixture over four bread slices, add Manchego cheese and cover with the top bread piece.

If you have a Panini maker, cook on it until you see the bread turning brown. If you don't have a Panini maker, take a grilling pan or a skillet and coat it well with cooking spray. Let it come up to medium heat then place the Panini inside it. Take a smaller saucepan and place it on top of the Panini to compress it.

Make sure to weigh the smaller saucepan down to really compress the sandwich. Cook for 3-4minutes and then remove weight and cook the other side for 2-3 minutes, using the same technique.

Serve:

Serve hot or cold with your favorite beverage.

Spinach and Roast Chicken Panini

Nutritional Value per Serving:

Calories: 420,

Carbohydrates: 29.6g

Cholesterol: 70mg

Fat: 10.3g

Saturated Fat: 2.8g

Sodium: 678mg

Protein: 26.4g

Fiber: 2.3g

Serving Size: 1

Preparation Time: 10 minutes

Cooking Time: 5 minutes

Ingredients:

Tomato	1 (sliced)
Deli roast chicken	½ cup (precooked and roughly chopped)
Mozzarella cheese	2 tbsp
Baby spinach	1 tbsp (chopped)
Onion	½ (sliced)
Basil pesto	According to taste
Sea salt and pepper	According to taste
Almond Oil	A few drops

Ciabatta roll	1 (cut lengthwise)

Method:

Lightly rub the roll with almond oil on both sides. Spread some basil pesto inside and then add all the ingredients with cheese on top. Cover with the other half of roll.

If you have a Panini maker, cook on it until you see the bread turning brown. If you don't have a Panini maker, take a grilling pan or a skillet and coat it well with cooking spray. Let it come up to medium heat then place the Panini inside it. Take a smaller saucepan and place it on top of the Panini to compress it.

Make sure to weigh the smaller saucepan down to really compress the sandwich. Cook for 3-4minutes and then remove weight and cook the other side for 2-3 minutes, using the same technique. Take out when golden brown.

Serve:

Serve hot or cold with your favorite beverage.

Roast Beef Panini

Nutritional Value per Serving:

Calories: 652

Carbohydrates: 77.3g

Cholesterol: 96mg

Fat: 23.3g

Saturated Fat: -

Sodium: 2113mg

Protein: 34.7g

Fiber: 3.1g

Serving Size: 6

Preparation Time: 10 minutes

Cooking Time: 15 minutes

Ingredients:

Unsalted butter	3 tbsp
Deli roast beef	1 pound (thinly sliced)
Large shallots	6 (sliced)
Cheese	1 cup (shredded)
Salt and pepper	According to taste
Mustard	2 tbsp
French baguettes	2 (cut lengthwise)

Method:

Heat butter over medium heat and add in shallots, cooking for 10 minutes or till tender. Add salt and pepper and set aside. Lay mustard on bread and add cheese on top. Then add roast beef, shallots and cover with bread pieces.

If you have a Panini maker, cook on it until you see the bread turning brown. If you don't have a Panini maker, take a grilling pan or a skillet and coat it well with cooking spray. Let it come up to medium heat then place the Panini inside it. Take a smaller saucepan and place it on top of the Panini to compress it.

Make sure to weigh the smaller saucepan down to really compress the sandwich. Cook for 3-4minutes and then remove weight and cook the other side for 2-3 minutes, using the same technique.

Serve:

Serve hot or cold with your favorite beverage.

Basil and Pepper Panini

Nutritional Value per Serving:

Calories: 290.6

Carbohydrates: 26.4g

Cholesterol: 40.9mg

Fat: 15g

Saturated Fat: 8.5g

Sodium: 642mg

Protein: 12.1g

Fiber: 1.4g

Serving Size: 4

Preparation Time: 10 minutes

Cooking Time: 5 minutes

Ingredients:

Mozzarella cheese	1 cup (shredded)
Roasted red peppers	4 whole (cut into strips)
Cheddar cheese	¼ cp (grated)
Basil leaves	15 (chopped)
Butter	2 tbsp
Italian Bread	8 slices

Method:

Heat up butter on medium heat and add 4 bread slices to it. Add pepper and both the cheeses. Top with other bread pieces and cook for about 2 minutes on both sides or until cheese melts.

If you have a Panini maker, cook on it until you see the bread turning brown. If you don't have a Panini maker, take a grilling pan or a skillet and coat it well with cooking spray. Let it come up to medium heat then place the Panini inside it. Take a smaller saucepan and place it on top of the Panini to compress it.

Make sure to weigh the smaller saucepan down to really compress the sandwich. Cook for 3-4minutes and then remove weight and cook the other side for 2-3 minutes, using the same technique.

Take out in a plate, sprinkle basil leaves on top and serve.

Serve:

Serve hot or cold with your favorite beverage.

Basil Pesto and Portobello Mushroom Panini

Nutritional Value per Serving:

Calories: 226

Carbohydrates: 15.5g

Cholesterol: 31.8mg

Fat: 12.9g

Saturated Fat: 7.8g

Sodium: 502.3mg

Protein: 14.4g

Fiber: 3.8g

Serving Size: 2

Preparation Time: 20 minutes

Cooking Time: 3 minutes

Ingredients:

Portobello mushrooms	4 (stems removed)
Basil pesto	2 tbsp
Ciabatta rolls	2
Balsamic vinegar	2 tbsp
Sea salt and pepper	According to taste
Almond oil	According to need
Taleggio cheese	3 1/2

Method:

Preheat grill on medium heat. Cut off the bottom and top sides of ciabatta rolls and cut them lengthwise. Pour pesto sauce in them and set aside.

Add a teaspoon of almond oil, vinegar, salt and pepper to mushrooms and grill for 2 minutes.

Add the mushrooms and cheese to rolls and put back in grill for 2 minutes each side or until golden brown.

If you have a Panini maker, cook on it until you see the bread turning brown. If you don't have a Panini maker, take a grilling pan or a skillet and coat it well with cooking spray. Let it come up to medium heat then place the Panini inside it. Take a smaller saucepan and place it on top of the Panini to compress it.

Make sure to weigh the smaller saucepan down to really compress the sandwich. Cook for 3-4minutes and then remove weight and cook the other side for 2-3 minutes, using the same technique.

Serve:

Serve hot or cold with your favorite beverage.

Beani Panini

Nutritional Value per Serving:

Calories: 209

Carbohydrates: 20.3g

Cholesterol: 80mg

Fat: 15.1g

Saturated Fat: 9.6g

Sodium: 602.8mg

Protein: 28g

Fiber: 5.2g

Serving Size: 1

Preparation Time: 12 minutes

Cooking Time: 6 minutes

Ingredients:

Cannellini beans	½ cup (drained)
Garlic powder	½ tsp
Sea salt and pepper	According to taste
Apple cider vinegar	2 tsp
Honey	½ tsp
Coconut oil	2 tsp
Cheese	2 tbsp
Sourdough bread	2 slices

Baby spinach	3 tbsp (shopped)

Method:

Mix together the first 6 ingredients, till coconut oil. Let marinate for 10-12 minutes. Then cook in the microwave for about 1-2 minutes and set aside. Heat up the grill on medium heat and toast the bread slices until warm. Add the bean mixture on top along with a tbsp of spinach. Sprinkle cheese on top, cover with bread slice and grill for 2 minutes on both sides.

If you have a Panini maker, cook on it until you see the bread turning brown. If you don't have a Panini maker, take a grilling pan or a skillet and coat it well with cooking spray. Let it come up to medium heat then place the Panini inside it. Take a smaller saucepan and place it on top of the Panini to compress it.

Make sure to weigh the smaller saucepan down to really compress the sandwich. Cook for 3-4minutes and then remove weight and cook the other side for 2-3 minutes, using the same technique.

Serve:

Serve hot or cold with your favorite beverage.

Classic Reuben Panini

Nutritional Value per Serving:

Calories: 500

Carbohydrates: 30g

Cholesterol: 100mg

Fat: 31g

Saturated Fat: 14g

Sodium: 1630mg

Protein: 23g

Fiber: 4g

Serving Size: 1

Preparation Time: 25 minutes

Cooking Time: 5 minutes

Ingredients:

Corned beef	½ pound (thinly sliced)
Butter	2 tbsp (softened)
Mozzarella cheese	8 slices
Any dressing of your choice	According to need
Sauerkraut	1 cup (drained and dried)
Sourdough bread	8 slices

Method:

Heat your skillet grill on medium heat. Spread butter on 4 slices of bread and dressing on the other 4. Add ¼ cup of sauerkraut on 4 bread slices, along with 2 ounces corned beef, 2 slices of cheese and cover with the top bread piece.

If you have a Panini maker, cook on it until you see the bread turning brown. If you don't have a Panini maker, take a grilling pan or a skillet and coat it well with cooking spray. Let it come up to medium heat then place the Panini inside it. Take a smaller saucepan and place it on top of the Panini to compress it.

Make sure to weigh the smaller saucepan down to really compress the sandwich. Cook for 3-4minutes and then remove weight and cook the other side for 2-3 minutes, using the same technique.

Serve:

Serve hot or cold with your favorite beverage.

Buffalo Chicken Panini

Nutritional Value per Serving:

Calories: 379

Carbohydrates: 41.2g

Cholesterol: 67mg

Fat: 11.8g

Saturated Fat: -

Sodium: 1496mg

Protein: 28.5g

Fiber: 1.5g

Serving Size: 4

Preparation Time: 20 minutes

Cooking Time: 5 minutes

Ingredients:

Cooked chicken	2 cups (shredded)
Feta cheese	1/3 cup (crumbled)
Italian loaf	1 (11 ounces)
Medium Buffalo wing sauce	½ cup

Method:

In a bowl, mix cooked chicken, buffalo wing sauce and microwave on high for 3 minutes. Cut the loaf in 8 rectangular pieces and grill on medium heat for 2 minutes each side. Take out and spread the chicken mixture on 4 bread pieces, add cheese on top and cover with other bread pieces. Put back in the grill and toast for another 2 minutes.

If you have a Panini maker, cook on it until you see the bread turning brown. If you don't have a Panini maker, take a grilling pan or a skillet and coat it well with cooking spray. Let it come up to medium heat then place the Panini inside it. Take a smaller saucepan and place it on top of the Panini to compress it.

Make sure to weigh the smaller saucepan down to really compress the sandwich. Cook for 3-4minutes and then remove weight and cook the other side for 2-3 minutes, using the same technique.

Serve:

Serve hot or cold with your favorite beverage.

Grilled Asparagus and Prosciutto Panini

Nutritional Value per Serving:

Calories: 215.2

Carbohydrates: 5.9g

Cholesterol: 44.8mg

Fat: 15.1g

Saturated Fat: 7.8g

Sodium: 372mg

Protein: 15.3g

Fiber: 2.2g

Serving Size: 4

Preparation Time: 10 minutes

Cooking Time: 5 minutes

Ingredients:

Prosciutto	4 slices
Asparagus	1 pound (ends broken)
Almond oil	2 tbsp
Mozzarella cheese	8 ounces
Sea salt and pepper	According to taste
Italian bread	4 pieces (sliced)

Method:

In a bowl, mix oil, salt and pepper in asparagus and mix well. Heat the grill on medium and cook asparagus for 3 minutes or till they get soft. Set aside. Clean the grill and heat on medium high.

On bread, place prosciutto, add ¼ of cheese and as many asparagus as you like. Top with the other slice and grill for 5 minutes till the cheese melts and starts running.

If you have a Panini maker, cook on it until you see the bread turning brown. If you don't have a Panini maker, take a grilling pan or a skillet and coat it well with cooking spray. Let it come up to medium heat then place the Panini inside it. Take a smaller saucepan and place it on top of the Panini to compress it.

Make sure to weigh the smaller saucepan down to really compress the sandwich. Cook for 3-4minutes and then remove weight and cook the other side for 2-3 minutes, using the same technique.

Serve:

Serve hot or cold with your favorite beverage.

Ham and Brie Panini

Nutritional Value per Serving:

Calories: 457

Carbohydrates: 42.7g

Cholesterol: 57mg

Fat: 24.5g

Saturated Fat: -

Sodium: 880mg

Protein: 16.8g

Fiber: 1.6g

Serving Size: 2

Preparation Time: 10 minutes

Cooking Time: 6 minutes

Ingredients:

Black forest ham	6 slices
Coconut oil	1 tbsp
Brie cheese	8 ounce (sliced)
Paleo mayonnaise	1 tbsp
Apricot preserves	2 tbsp
Italia bread	4 slices

Method:

On 2 bread slices, spread apricot preserves, ham, brie and mayo and cover with the other two slices.

Take a smaller saucepan and place it on top of the Panini to compress it. Brush some oil on top and bottom of the sandwich.

If you have a Panini maker, cook on it until you see the bread turning brown. If you don't have a Panini maker, take a grilling pan or a skillet and coat it well with cooking spray. Let it come up to medium heat then place the Panini inside it. Take a smaller saucepan and place it on top of the Panini to compress it.

Make sure to weigh the smaller saucepan down to really compress the sandwich. Cook for 3-4minutes and then remove weight and cook the other side for 2-3 minutes, using the same technique.

Serve:

Serve hot or cold with your favorite beverage.

Nutritional Value per Serving:

Calories: 710

Carbohydrates: 42g

Cholesterol: 522mg

Fat: 44g

Saturated Fat: 22g

Sodium: 1510mg

Protein: 36g

Fiber: 3g

Serving Size: 4

Preparation Time: 25 minutes

Cooking Time: 5 minutes

Ingredients:

Ciabatta bread	1 loaf (thinly sliced)
Fontina cheese	6 ounces (sliced)
Bell peppers	4 (roasted)
Caramelized onion marmalade	¾ cup
Fresh basil	1 bunch
Cooked chicken	1 pound (slightly shredded)
Kalamata olives	4 ounces (pitted)
Artichoke hearts	4 ounces (marinated)

| Basil leaves | 2 (fresh) |
| Thyme leaves | 1 teaspoon (fresh) |

Method:

Take the olives, the artichoke hearts, basil and thyme leaves and pulse them together in the food processor until they are all coarsely chopped and mixed together.

Take some ciabatta bread and spread the olive tapenade on the slices according to your tastes. Add on the cheese and the roasted peppers. Add some shredded chicken and basil leaves and spread a tablespoon of some caramelized onion jam on the last slice.

If you have a Panini maker, cook on it until you see the bread turning brown. If you don't have a Panini maker, take a grilling pan or a skillet and coat it well with cooking spray. Let it come up to medium heat then place the Panini inside it. Take a smaller saucepan and place it on top of the Panini to compress it.

Make sure to weigh the smaller saucepan down to really compress the sandwich. Cook for 3-4minutes and then remove weight and cook the other side for 2-3 minutes, using the same technique.

Serve:

Serve hot or cold with your favorite beverage.

Braised Short Rib Panini

Nutritional Value per Serving:

Calories: 380

Carbohydrates: 3.0g

Cholesterol: 85 mg

Fat: 31.9g

Saturated Fat: 13.1g

Sodium: 350mg

Protein: 20g

Fiber: 0.0g

Serving Size: 4

Preparation Time: 25 minutes

Cooking Time: 5 minutes

Ingredients:

Sourdough bread	12 slices
Balsamic onion marmalade	¾ cup
Braised short ribs	4 cups (shredded)
Aged Cheddar	12 ounces (shredded)
Butter	2 tablespoons (melted)

Method:

Take some sourdough bread and add a generous amount of the shredded braised short rib meat and caramelized onion. Top off with almost ¼ cup of cheddar cheese and add the other slice on top to close the sandwich. Brush with the some melted butter before you start to grill the sandwiches

If you have a Panini maker, cook on it until you see the bread turning brown. If you don't have a Panini maker, take a grilling pan or a skillet and coat it well with cooking spray. Let it come up to medium heat then place the Panini inside it. Take a smaller saucepan and place it on top of the Panini to compress it.

Make sure to weigh the smaller saucepan down to really compress the sandwich. Cook for 3-4minutes and then remove weight and cook the other side for 2-3 minutes, using the same technique.

Serve:

Serve hot or cold with your favorite beverage.

Green Chile Steak Melt Panini

Nutritional Value per Serving:

Calories: 380

Carbohydrates: 3.0g

Cholesterol: 85 mg

Fat: 31.9g

Saturated Fat: 13.1g

Sodium: 350mg

Protein: 20g

Fiber: 0.0g

Serving Size: 4

Preparation Time: 15 minutes

Cooking Time: 35 minutes

Ingredients:

Ciabatta bread	1 loaf
Extra virgin olive oil	1 tablespoon
Chipotle mayonnaise	According to taste
Strip steak	1 pound
Monetary Jack Cheese	8 slices
Caramelized onions	¾ cup
Roasted green chiles	17 oz can (chopped)
Salt and Pepper	According to taste

Method:

Heat a skillet and bring it up to a moderately high heat. While it's heating, season the steak with salt and pepper and let it sit for a bit. Add some olive oil in the pan and add the steak to cook as well. Make sure to cook the steak till you get your level of preferred cooked meat.

Rest the steak for 10 minutes before cutting into thin slices, crosswise. Take some bread and spread around a tablespoon of mayonnaise on one slice. Add some cheese, onions, steak, the chiles and another slice of cheese. Add another slice of bread and apply some mayonnaise on it before adding it on.

If you have a Panini maker, cook on it until you see the bread turning brown. If you don't have a Panini maker, take a grilling pan or a skillet and coat it well with cooking spray. Let it come up to medium heat then place the Panini inside it. Take a smaller saucepan and place it on top of the Panini to compress it.

Make sure to weigh the smaller saucepan down to really compress the sandwich. Cook for 3-4minutes and then remove weight and cook the other side for 2-3 minutes, using the same technique.

Serve:

Serve hot or cold with your favorite beverage.

Prosciutto Wrapped Turkey and Avocado Panini

Nutritional Value per Serving:

Calories: 720

Carbohydrates: 53.1g

Cholesterol: 125 mg

Fat: 31.9g

Saturated Fat: 13.1g

Sodium: 1650mg

Protein: 25.8g

Fiber: 2.8g

Serving Size: 2

Preparation Time: 10 minutes

Cooking Time: 5 minutes

Ingredients:

Ciabatta bread	4 slices (You can substitute with Pugliese)
Sun dried tomatoes	2 tablespoons (chopped)
Mayonnaise	3 tablespoons
Prosciutto	2 slices
Turkey breast	2 slices (large, roasted)
Avocado	½ avocados (thinly sliced)
Swiss Cheese	4 slices
Salt and Pepper	According to taste

Method:

Preheat a skillet to medium-high heat. Take a small bowl and mix the sun dried tomatoes with the mayonnaise. Spread the mixture evenly on one side of all the slices. Now add a slice of Swiss cheese, wrap the prosciutto around the turkey and place it on top of the Swiss cheese. Add a slice of avocado, another slice of Swiss cheese and top off with the remaining slice of bread.

Rest the steak for 10 minutes before cutting into thin slices, crosswise. Take some bread and spread around a tablespoon of mayonnaise on one slice. Add some cheese, onions, steak, the chiles and another slice of cheese. Add another slice of bread and apply some mayonnaise on it before adding it on.

If you have a Panini maker, cook on it until you see the bread turning brown. If you don't have a Panini maker, take a grilling pan or a skillet and coat it well with cooking spray. Let it come up to medium heat then place the Panini inside it. Take a smaller saucepan and place it on top of the Panini to compress it.

Make sure to weigh the smaller saucepan down to really compress the sandwich. Cook for 3-4minutes and then remove weight and cook the other side for 2-3 minutes, using the same technique. Grill for 5-6 minutes or until golden brown and the cheese starts to melt.

Serve:

Serve hot or cold with your favorite beverage.

Red Chile Chicken Panini

Nutritional Value per Serving:

Calories: 280

Carbohydrates: 23.0g

Cholesterol: 50 mg

Fat: 117g

Saturated Fat: 7.0g

Sodium: 350mg

Protein: 20g

Fiber: 0.0g

Serving Size: 4

Preparation Time: 45 minutes

Cooking Time: 35 minutes

Ingredients:

Sour dough bread	8 slices
Olive oil	1 tablespoon
Mexican red chile sauce	1¼ cup
White vinegar	2 tablespoons (can be substituted with cider vinegar)
Cloves	½ teaspoon (grounded)
All spice	½ teaspoon (grounded)
Cinnamon	1 teaspoon
Cumin	¼ teaspoon (grounded)

Dried oregano	a pinch (crushed)
Garlic	1 teaspoon (minced)
Chicken thighs	6 (boneless, skinless)
Red onion	1 (thinly sliced)
Avocado	1 (thinly sliced)
Monterey jack cheese	4-6 oz.
Butter	2 tablespoons (melted)
Mayonnaise	According to taste
Salt and Pepper	According to taste

Method:

Take a medium sized pan and heat some oil in it before adding the chile sauce to it. Add in the cumin, all spice, cinnamon, cloves, vinegar, oregano, garlic and pepper. Bring to a simmer and simmer for 5 minutes before setting it aside to cool.

Apply salt on both sides of the chicken thighs. Take a zip lock baggie or a non-reactive bowl and mix the chicken with the marinade once it cools down. Let it stay in the refrigerator for 30 minutes or longer.*

Take the chicken out of the refrigerator and then start preheating a grill to medium-high heat. Brush some olive oil on the grill and cook the chicken for 3-4 minutes on each side.

Now take the melted butter and brush it on the outer side of each bread slice. Spread a thin, even layer on the bottom slice and add the onions, cheese, avocado and 1-2 chicken thighs. Top off with the other slice of bread and make sure that it is buttered side up.

If you have a Panini maker, cook on it until you see the bread turning brown. If you don't have a Panini maker, take a grilling pan or a skillet and coat it well with cooking spray. Let it come up to medium heat then place the Panini inside it. Take a smaller saucepan and place it on top of the Panini to compress it.

Make sure to weigh the smaller saucepan down to really compress the sandwich. Cook for 3-4minutes and then remove weight and cook the other side for 2-3 minutes, using the same technique.

Serve:

Serve hot or cold with your favorite beverage.

*Note:

Remember, the longer you marinade something, the better it tastes so leaving the chicken to marinade for an hour or to marinade overnight can be a good idea too.

Spinach and Chicken Panini with Lemon Herbs
Nutritional Value per Serving:

Calories: 300

Carbohydrates: 40.0g

Cholesterol: 30 mg

Fat: 63g

Saturated Fat: 2.0g

Sodium: 600mg

Protein: 20.0g

Fiber: 5.0g

Serving Size: 3

Preparation Time: 15 minutes

Cooking Time: 25 minutes

Ingredients:

Ciabatta bread	6 slices
Chicken breasts	½ lb (boneless, skinless)
Spinach	1 8oz. packet (frozen, chopped)
Salt	¼ teaspoon
Pepper	1/8 teaspoon
Rosemary	½ teaspoon (dried)
Parsley	½ teaspoon (dried)
Thyme	¼ teaspoon (dried)

Lemon	1
Olive oil	for brushing only
Pesto paste	any will do. For spreading only
Sun dried tomatoes	1 can (drained and julienned)
Parmesan cheese	2 cups (shredded or shaved)

Method:

Preheat your grill to medium high heat. Now take a small bowl and mix together the rosemary, salt, pepper, thyme and parsley. Once they're all mixed, take the chicken breasts and press the herb rub on both sides of the chicken. Cut the lemon in half and squeeze out the juice on top of the chicken breasts. Put the chicken on the grill and cook for 6-7 minutes or until it's cooked through.

Brush a little olive oil on the outer sides of the bread. Spread a thin layer of the pesto paste on the inside of the bread. Add on enough spinach to cover the slice completely. Take the chicken breasts and slice each into strips. Place 4-5 strips on top of the spinach and sprinkle some sun-dried tomatoes and a generous helping of Parmesan cheese on top of the chicken.

If you have a Panini maker, cook on it until you see the bread turning brown. If you don't have a Panini maker, take a grilling pan or a skillet and coat it well with cooking spray. Let it come up to medium heat then place the Panini inside it. Take a smaller saucepan and place it on top of the Panini to compress it. Make sure to weigh the smaller saucepan down to really compress the sandwich. Cook for 3-4minutes and then remove weight and cook the other side for 2-3 minutes, using the same technique.

Serve:

Serve hot or cold with your favorite beverage.

Barbecued Salmon Panini
Nutritional Value per Serving:

Calories: 230

Carbohydrates: 9.0g

Cholesterol: 85 mg

Fat: 11g

Saturated Fat: 1.5g

Sodium: 530mg

Protein: 24.0g

Fiber: 1.0g

Serving Size: 4

Preparation Time: 15 minutes

Cooking Time: 25 minutes

Ingredients:

Mayonnaise	1 cup
Barbecue sauce	1 cup
Green onion	1(chopped)
Celery	2 tablespoons (minced)
Parsley	2 tablespoons (fresh, chopped)
Garlic	1 clove (minced)
Fresh Salmon	1 lb
Panko bread crumbs	1 cup
Canola oil	for brushing only

Rustic bread	8 slices
Red onion	1 (thinly sliced)
Tomatoes	2 (thinly sliced)
Salt and Pepper	According to taste

Method:

Combine the barbeque sauce and mayonnaise in a medium sized bowl. Once they're mixed well, add in the parsley, celery, garlic and onion. Season well with salt and pepper and refrigerate until needed.

Divide the salmon into 4 portions equally. Brush the top and sides of the salmon with the barbeque sauce and coat with panko crumbs. Oil up the grill and cook the salmon, skin side down for 8-10 minutes or until completely cooked through. Take the barbeque remoulade and spread it generously on the bread. Layer with some red onion, salmon and tomatoes then close the sandwich with the other slice of bread.

If you have a Panini maker, cook on it until you see the bread turning brown. If you don't have a Panini maker, take a grilling pan or a skillet and coat it well with cooking spray. Let it come up to medium heat then place the Panini inside it. Take a smaller saucepan and place it on top of the Panini to compress it.

Make sure to weigh the smaller saucepan down to really compress the sandwich. Cook for 3-4minutes and then remove weight and cook the other side for 2-3 minutes, using the same technique.

Serve:

Serve hot or cold with your favorite beverage.

Crispy Fish Panini

Nutritional Value per Serving:

Calories: 230

Carbohydrates: 9.0g

Cholesterol: 85 mg

Fat: 11g

Saturated Fat: 1.5g

Sodium: 530mg

Protein: 24.0g

Fiber: 1.0g

Serving Size: 4

Preparation Time: 15 minutes

Cooking Time: 25 minutes

Ingredients:

Tartar sauce	3 cups
Fish patties	4
Cheddar cheese	3 oz. (grated)
English muffins	4

Method:

Cut the English muffin into half and spread a generous amount of tartar sauce on the bottom half of it. Place a fish patty on top and sprinkle on some cheddar cheese. Add on the other half of the muffin and grill for 7-8 minutes or until the cheese starts to melt.

If you have a Panini maker, cook on it until you see the bread turning brown. If you don't have a Panini maker, take a grilling pan or a skillet and coat it well with cooking spray. Let it come up to medium heat then place the Panini inside it. Take a smaller saucepan and place it on top of the Panini to compress it.

Make sure to weigh the smaller saucepan down to really compress the sandwich. Cook for 3-4minutes and then remove weight and cook the other side for 2-3 minutes, using the same technique.

Serve:

Serve hot or cold with your favorite beverage.

Mango and Avocado Panini with Grilled Crabs

Nutritional Value per Serving:

Calories: 650

Carbohydrates: 48g

Cholesterol: 85 mg

Fat: 36g

Saturated Fat: 14.0g

Sodium: 2610mg

Protein: 34.0g

Fiber: 1.0g

Serving Size: 4

Preparation Time: 15 minutes

Cooking Time: 15 minutes

Ingredients:

Crab meat	12 oz. (fresh, drained)
Lime juice	3 tablespoons (freshly squeezed)
French bread	8 (1/2 inch thick slices)
Butter	¼ cup (melted)
Avocados	2 (sliced)
Mango	1 (thinly sliced)
Muenster cheese	4 oz. (thinly sliced)
Black pepper	1/8 teaspoon (freshly ground)

Method:

Combine the pepper, the crab and lime juice together in a small bowl and set aside. Take the bread and brush the outer sides with butter. Place the avocado slices, the crab mixture, some mango slices and sprinkle on with cheese before closing with the other bread slice.

If you have a Panini maker, cook on it until you see the bread turning brown. If you don't have a Panini maker, take a grilling pan or a skillet and coat it well with cooking spray. Let it come up to medium heat then place the Panini inside it. Take a smaller saucepan and place it on top of the Panini to compress it.

Make sure to weigh the smaller saucepan down to really compress the sandwich. Cook for 3-4minutes and then remove weight and cook the other side for 2-3 minutes, using the same technique.

Serve:

Serve hot or cold with your favorite beverage.

Heirloom Tomato Panini

Nutritional Value per Serving:

Calories: 146

Carbohydrates: 8.0g

Cholesterol: 14mg

Fat: 11g

Saturated Fat: 3.0g

Sodium: 221mg

Protein: 5.0g

Fiber: 1.0g

Serving Size: 4

Preparation Time: 15 minutes

Cooking Time: 15 minutes

Ingredients:

Heirloom tomatoes	2 (sliced thinly)
Lime juice	3 tablespoons (freshly squeezed)
Sour dough bread	8 slices
Mayonnaise	¼ cup
Salt and Pepper	According to taste

Method:

Spread the mayonnaise as thickly as you like on the bread. Add some tomato slices and season them with salt and pepper. Close the sandwich by placing the bread mayonnaise side down.

If you have a Panini maker, cook on it until you see the bread turning brown. If you don't have a Panini maker, take a grilling pan or a skillet and coat it well with cooking spray. Let it come up to medium heat then place the Panini inside it. Take a smaller saucepan and place it on top of the Panini to compress it.

Make sure to weigh the smaller saucepan down to really compress the sandwich. Cook for 1-2minutes and then remove weight and cook the other side for 1-2 minutes, using the same technique.

Serve:

Serve hot or cold with your favorite beverage.

Avocado and Mashed Chickpea Panini

Nutritional Value per Serving:

Calories: 352

Carbohydrates: 14.3g

Cholesterol: 85 mg

Fat: 11g

Saturated Fat: 14.0g

Sodium: 621mg

Protein: 14.3g

Fiber: 14g

Serving Size: 4

Preparation Time: 20 minutes

Cooking Time: 10 minutes

Ingredients:

Chickpeas	1 can (15 ounce, drained, peeled, rinsed)
Avocado	1 large (ripe, pitted, quartered and peeled)
Basil	2 tablespoons (chopped)
Italian parsley	2 tablespoons (chopped)
Scallions	2 tablespoons
Lemon juice	2 (freshly squeezed)
Basil pesto	4 tablespoons
Red bell peppers	¼ cup (roasted)

Butter	4 tablespoons (room temperature)
Salt and Pepper	According to taste
Asiago	4ounces (can be substituted with other sharp cheese)

Method:

Take a medium sized bowl and mash the chickpeas and avocado chunks together until you get a chunky texture. Mix in the scallions, lemon juice, parsley and basil and season with some salt and pepper.

Spread butter on the outside of the slices. Flip them over and spread basil pesto on the inside. Add a slice of cheese and then spoon a generous helping of the avocado and chickpea mixture. Add a roasted pepper on top and another slice of cheese before closing the sandwich and grilling it.

If you have a Panini maker, cook on it until you see the bread turning brown. If you don't have a Panini maker, take a grilling pan or a skillet and coat it well with cooking spray. Let it come up to medium heat then place the Panini inside it. Take a smaller saucepan and place it on top of the Panini to compress it.

Make sure to weigh the smaller saucepan down to really compress the sandwich. Cook for 1-2minutes and then remove weight and cook the other side for 1-2 minutes, using the same technique.

Serve:

Serve hot or cold with your favorite beverage.

Wild Mushroom Melt Panini
Nutritional Value per Serving:

Calories: 460

Carbohydrates: 62.0g

Cholesterol: 20 mg

Fat: 14g

Saturated Fat: 14.0g

Sodium: 1310 mg

Protein: 9.0g

Fiber: 4.0g

Serving Size: 4

Preparation Time: 10 minutes

Cooking Time: 20 minutes

Ingredients:

Extra virgin olive oil	1 tablespoon
Unsalted Butter	1 tablespoon
Shallots	¼ cup (thinly sliced)
Garlic	2 teaspoons (minced)
Scallions	2 tablespoons
Wild mushrooms	2 ½ cup (sliced, shitake, porcini or chanterelle)
Balsamic vinegar	1 tablespoon
Parsley	1 tablespoon (chopped)
Salt and Pepper	According to taste
Swiss cheese	½ pound (can be substituted with other sharp cheese)
Rye bread	8 slices
Butter	4 tablespoons

Method:

Combine the olive oil and unsalted butter in a skillet on medium heat until they melt. Add in the garlic and shallots and cook until they become fragrant or for a minute. Now add the mushrooms and cook for 5-7 minutes, stirring occasionally or until the mushrooms grow tender. Add the parsley and balsamic vinegar as well as salt and pepper.

Spread the butter on the outside of the bread. On the inside of the bread, place a slice of cheese, some sautéed mushrooms and top off with some more cheese. Add the other slice of bread and close the sandwich, making sure that the buttered side is outside.

If you have a Panini maker, cook on it until you see the bread turning brown. If you don't have a Panini maker, take a grilling pan or a skillet and coat it well with cooking spray. Let it come up to medium heat then place the Panini inside it. Take a smaller saucepan and place it on top of the Panini to compress it.

Make sure to weigh the smaller saucepan down to really compress the sandwich. Cook for 1-2minutes and then remove weight and cook the other side for 1-2 minutes, using the same technique.

Serve:

Serve hot or cold with your favorite beverage.

BBQ Chicken Panini
Nutritional Value per Serving:

Calories: 259

Carbohydrates: 32.0g

Cholesterol: 0 mg

Fat: 10g

Saturated Fat: 1.0g

Sodium: 742 mg

Protein: 12.0g

Fiber: 5.0g

Serving Size: 4

Preparation Time: 10 minutes

Cooking Time: 15 minutes

Ingredients:

Onion	¼ cup (thinly sliced)
Chicken breasts	2-3 lbs (boneless, skinless)
Canola oil	1 tablespoon
Barbeque sauce	½ cup
Cabbage	1½ cup tablespoons
Mayonnaise	2 tablespoons (can use low fat)
Red wine vinegar	2 teaspoons
Garlic powder	¼ teaspoon
Salt and Pepper	According to taste
Dill pickles	½ pound (can be substituted with other sharp cheese)
Rye bread	8 slices
Butter	4 tablespoons

Method:

Soak the onion in cold water in a small bowl and set aside. Heat the oil on medium heat in a non-stick skillet. Add the chicken breasts and cook for four minutes on each side or until they start to turn brown. Bring the heat down to low and add in the barbeque sauce. Make sure to coat the chicken breasts in the sauce, cover it and cook on low heat for 3 minutes more.

In a separate bowl, combine the vinegar, cabbage, garlic powder, salt and pepper and toss well. Drain the onions. Take some butter and apply it on the outside of the bread. Place about 1/3 cup of the coleslaw on the bun then top off with a chicken breast, a dill pickle and some onions. If there's any sauce in the pan, smear that on top and then close the sandwich with a slice of bread.

If you have a Panini maker, cook on it until you see the bread turning brown. If you don't have a Panini maker, take a grilling pan or a skillet and coat it well with cooking spray. Let it come up to medium heat then place the Panini inside it. Take a smaller saucepan and place it on top of the Panini to compress it.

Make sure to weigh the smaller saucepan down to really compress the sandwich. Cook for 1-2minutes and then remove weight and cook the other side for 1-2 minutes, using the same technique.

Serve:

Serve hot or cold with your favorite beverage.

Italian Grilled Pork Panini

Nutritional Value per Serving:

Calories: 454

Carbohydrates: 32.0g

Cholesterol: 75 mg

Fat: 22g

Saturated Fat: 5.0g

Sodium: 690 mg

Protein: 32.0g

Fiber: 5.0g

Serving Size: 4

Preparation Time: 10 minutes

Cooking Time: 10 minutes

Ingredients:

Pork chops	6 (cooked, sliced thinly)
Pesto	½ cup
Italian bread	8 slices
Provolone cheese	4 slices
Olive oil	1 tablespoon (for brushing only)

Method:

Spread the pesto on the on every slice of bread. Top off with some slices of pork chops and add the cheese on top. Close the sandwich with the remaining bread slices and brush with some olive oil.

If you have a Panini maker, cook on it until you see the bread turning brown. If you don't have a Panini maker, take a grilling pan or a skillet and coat it well with cooking spray. Let it come up to medium heat then place the Panini inside it. Take a smaller saucepan and place it on top of the Panini to compress it.

Make sure to weigh the smaller saucepan down to really compress the sandwich. Cook for 1-2minutes and then remove weight and cook the other side for 1-2 minutes, using the same technique.

Serve:

Serve hot or cold with your favorite beverage.

Egg and Salmon Panini
Nutritional Value per Serving:

Calories: 214

Carbohydrates: 25.0g

Cholesterol: 7 mg

Fat: 5g

Saturated Fat: 1.0g

Sodium: 670 mg

Protein: 19.0g

Fiber: 3.0g

Serving Size: 1

Preparation Time: 15 minutes

Cooking Time: 15 minutes

Ingredients:

Extra virgin olive oil	½ teaspoon
Red onion	1 tablespoon (finely chopped)
Egg whites	2 (large, beaten)
Capers	½ teaspoon (chopped, rinsed)
Smoked salmon	1 ounce
Tomato	1 (sliced)
Sourdough bread	2 slices
Salt and Pepper	According to taste

Method:

Over medium heat, take a large non-stick skillet and heat some oil. Add the onions to it and cook for 1 minute or until they start to soften. Add the capers, egg whites and salt and cook while stirring constantly for 30 seconds or until the egg whites set.

Take some bread and layer with a generous helping of the egg white mixture. Add some smoked salmon, tomato and season a bit before closing the sandwich off.

If you have a Panini maker, cook on it until you see the bread turning brown. If you don't have a Panini maker, take a grilling pan or a skillet and coat it well with cooking spray. Let it come up to medium heat then place the Panini inside it. Take a smaller saucepan and place it on top of the Panini to compress it.

Make sure to weigh the smaller saucepan down to really compress the sandwich. Cook for 1-2minutes and then remove weight and cook the other side for 1-2 minutes, using the same technique.

Serve:

Serve hot or cold with your favorite beverage.

BLT (Bacon, Lettuce and Tomato) Panini

Nutritional Value per Serving:

Calories: 363

Carbohydrates: 46.0g

Cholesterol: 4 mg

Fat: 9g

Saturated Fat: 1.0g

Sodium: 670 mg

Protein: 17.0g

Fiber: 4.0g

Serving Size: 1

Preparation Time: 25 minutes

Cooking Time: 25 minutes

Ingredients:

Djon mustard	1 tablespoon
Soy sauce	1 tablespoon (reduced sodium)
Adobo sauce	1 teaspoon
Bacon	4 strips
Mayonnaise	4 tablespoons (can use low fat)
Ciabatta bread	8 slices
Lettuce	4 pieces (green leaf)

Tomatoes	2 (medium, sliced)
Salt and Pepper	According to taste

Method:

Preheat an oven at 475F. Take a medium sized bowl and mix the soy sauce, ½ teaspoon of adobo sauce and the mustard together. Take the bacon strips and bake in the oven for 20 minutes or until they become crispy.

In another bowl, mix the mayonnaise and the ½ teaspoon of adobo sauce. Spread on the bread. Take out the bacon and put 4 strips on the bread and add the tomato and lettuce as well. Close the sandwich and grill lightly to toast the bread.

If you have a Panini maker, cook on it until you see the bread turning brown. If you don't have a Panini maker, take a grilling pan or a skillet and coat it well with cooking spray. Let it come up to medium heat then place the Panini inside it. Take a smaller saucepan and place it on top of the Panini to compress it.

Make sure to weigh the smaller saucepan down to really compress the sandwich. Cook for 1-2minutes and then remove weight and cook the other side for 1-2 minutes, using the same technique.

Serve:

Serve hot or cold with your favorite beverage.

Mediterranean Melt Panini
Nutritional Value per Serving:

Calories: 290

Carbohydrates: 35.0g

Cholesterol: 5mg

Fat: 7g

Saturated Fat: 3.0g

Sodium: 440 mg

Protein: 21.0g

Fiber: 5.0g

Serving Size: 4

Preparation Time: 10 minutes

Cooking Time: 15 minutes

Ingredients:

Garlic clove	1 (large, finely grated or pasted)
Lemon	1 (juiced)
Extra virgin olive oil	3 tablespoons
Fresh thyme	a few sprigs (finely chopped)
Tuna	2 cans (6 ounce, line caught or Italian, drained)
Ciabatta bread	8 slices
Red onion	½ (small, chopped finely)
Capers	3 tablespoons (finely chopped)
Swiss cheese	4 slices
Plum tomatoes	2 (sliced thinly, lengthwise)
Parsley leaves	2 handfuls (can use baby arugula or celery tops too)
Provolone cheese	4 slices
Salt and Pepper	According to taste

Method:

Take a medium sized bowl and combine the olive oil, lemon juice, garlic, black pepper and thyme. Allow it to stand for a bit before adding in the capers, tuna and red onions. Mash everything to combine them.

Take some bread and add the Swiss cheese on 4 slices. Now add the tuna mix, greens, tomatoes and add the provolone cheese on top before closing off with the other slice of bread.

If you have a Panini maker, cook on it until you see the bread turning brown. If you don't have a Panini maker, take a grilling pan or a skillet and coat it well with cooking spray. Let it come up to medium heat then place the Panini inside it. Take a smaller saucepan and place it on top of the Panini to compress it.

Make sure to weigh the smaller saucepan down to really compress the sandwich. Cook for 1-2minutes and then remove weight and cook the other side for 1-2 minutes, using the same technique.

Serve:

Serve hot or cold with your favorite beverage.

Muffeletta Panini

Nutritional Value per Serving:

Calories: 838

Carbohydrates: 35.0g

Cholesterol: 154.4mg

Fat: 55g

Saturated Fat: 28.2g

Sodium: 2843.9 mg

Protein: 52.4g

Fiber: 1.7g

Serving Size: 4

Preparation Time: 10 minutes

Cooking Time: 5 minutes

Ingredients:

Butter	1 stick (softened)
Garlic clove	1 (large, finely grated or pasted)
Lemon	1 (juiced)
Extra virgin olive oil	3 tablespoons
Fresh thyme	a few sprigs (finely chopped)
Olive salad	½ cup (you can also use olive tapenade)
Sourdough bread	8 slices
Provolone cheese	16 slices
Black forest ham	6 ounces (sliced thinly)
Genoa salami	6 ounces (thinly sliced)
Mortadella	6 ounces (sliced)
Salt and Pepper	According to taste

Method:

Brush the bread with the butter and make sure it's on both sides. Layer the cheese over the 4 slices of bread. Top off with some ham, olive salad, salami, and the remaining cheese. Close the sandwich and put it on the grill.

If you have a Panini maker, cook on it until you see the bread turning brown. If you don't have a Panini maker, take a grilling pan or a skillet and coat it well with cooking spray.

Let it come up to medium heat then place the Panini inside it. Take a smaller saucepan and place it on top of the Panini to compress it.

Make sure to weigh the smaller saucepan down to really compress the sandwich. Cook for 1-2minutes and then remove weight and cook the other side for 1-2 minutes, using the same technique.

Serve:

Serve hot or cold with your favorite beverage.

Pickled Onion Salad with Patty Melt Panini

Nutritional Value per Serving:

Calories: 146

Carbohydrates: 8.0g

Cholesterol: 14mg

Fat: 11g

Saturated Fat: 3.0g

Sodium: 221mg

Protein: 5.0g

Fiber: 1.0g

Serving Size: 4

Preparation Time: 15 minutes

Cooking Time: 15 minutes

Ingredients:

Extra virgin olive oil	4 tablespoons
Yellow onions	4 (medium, halved, chopped lengthwise)

Rye bread	8 slices
Fresh Oregano	2 tablespoons (chopped)
Gruyere cheese	8 oz. (grated)
Salt and Pepper	According to taste

Method:

Cook the onions in a skillet with olive oil and stir constantly to avoid scorching them. Sprinkle on the oregano, salt and pepper and cook the onions until they start turning a deep brown or until they soften.

Take ¼ of the cheese and place it on the bread slice. Heap a generous amount of onions in and then close the sandwich.

If you have a Panini maker, cook on it until you see the bread turning brown. If you don't have a Panini maker, take a grilling pan or a skillet and coat it well with cooking spray. Let it come up to medium heat then place the Panini inside it. Take a smaller saucepan and place it on top of the Panini to compress it.

Make sure to weigh the smaller saucepan down to really compress the sandwich. Cook for 1-2minutes and then remove weight and cook the other side for 1-2 minutes, using the same technique.

Serve:

Serve hot or cold with your favorite beverage.

Grilled Vegetable Panini
Nutritional Value per Serving:

Calories: 146

Carbohydrates: 27g

Cholesterol: 9 mg

Fat: 20g

Saturated Fat: 2.0g

Sodium: 414mg

Protein: 5.0g

Fiber: 3.0g

Serving Size: 2

Preparation Time: 35 minutes

Cooking Time: 15 minutes

Ingredients:

Balsamic vinaigrette	According to taste
Japanese eggplant	1 (cut lengthwise)
Zucchini	1 (cut lengthwise)
Yellow onion	1 (sliced into rings)
Extra virgin olive oil	2 tablespoons
Olive bread	4 slices
Red peppers	2 (roasted)
Provolone cheese	4 slices
Hummus	According to taste
Salt and Pepper	According to taste

Method:

Marinate the zucchini and the eggplant in the balsamic vinaigrette for 20 minutes or more. Put them inside a zip lock baggie and chill in the refrigerator. Brush the onions on both sides with the olive oil and season them well with the salt and pepper. Place them on the grill. Take the zucchini and eggplant out of the marinade and put them on the grill as well. Cook them for 3-4 minutes on the grill.

Take some bread and layer some hummus on it. Add the zucchini, eggplant, red pepper, cheese, onion and close the sandwich. Brush with olive oil and then put on the grill.

If you have a Panini maker, cook on it until you see the bread turning brown. If you don't have a Panini maker, take a grilling pan or a skillet and coat it well with cooking spray. Let it come up to medium heat then place the Panini inside it. Take a smaller saucepan and place it on top of the Panini to compress it.

Make sure to weigh the smaller saucepan down to really compress the sandwich. Cook for 1-2minutes and then remove weight and cook the other side for 1-2 minutes, using the same technique.

Serve:

Serve hot or cold with your favorite beverage.

Caesar Shrimp and Arugula Panini
Nutritional Value per Serving:

Calories: 265

Carbohydrates: 28.9g

Cholesterol: 36mg

Fat: 9.7g

Saturated Fat: 5g

Sodium: 722mg

Protein: 14.5g

Fiber: 1.5g

Serving Size: 2

Preparation Time: 15 minutes

Cooking Time: 15 minutes

Ingredients

Large shrimps	¾ pound (peeled, de-veined)
Extra virgin olive oil	5 tablespoons
Fresh lemon juice	2 tablespoons
Garlic clove	1 (mashed through a garlic press)
Flat anchovies	2 (mashed)
Dijon mustard	1 teaspoon
Ciabtta rolls	2 (split in half
Arugula	1 cup (washed and dried)
Parmesan cheese	1 ounce (grated or shaved)
Salt and Pepper	According to taste

Method:

Season the shrimps with salt and pepper before tossing them well in olive oil. Put them on the grill and cook them for 2-3 minutes before setting aside to cool a bit.

Now combine the lemon juice, ¼ cup olive oil, anchovies, garlic and mustard in a medium sized bowl. Add the shrimps and mix well until they're well dressed in the mixture. Take the arugula rolls and layer the bottom half with some arugula, add the shrimps on top of the arugula and drizzle any remaining dressing sauce on them.

Add on the cheese and the top half of the roll before brushing with olive oil and putting it on the grill

If you have a Panini maker, cook on it until you see the cheese starting to melt and the bread turning brown.

If you don't have a Panini maker, take a grilling pan or a skillet and coat it well with cooking spray. Let it come up to medium heat then place the Panini inside it. Take a smaller saucepan and place it on top of the Panini to compress it.

Make sure to weigh the smaller saucepan down to really compress the sandwich. Cook for 3-4minutes and then remove weight and cook the other side for 2-3 minutes, using the same technique.

Serve:

Serve hot or cold with your favorite beverage.

Salmon Salad Panini

Nutritional Value per Serving:

Calories: 286

Carbohydrates: 29g

Cholesterol: 34mg

Fat: 9 g

Saturated Fat: 3g

Sodium: 645mg

Protein: 22g

Fiber: 4g

Serving Size: 4

Preparation Time: 15 minutes

Cooking Time: 15 minutes

Ingredients

Salmon	2 cans (6 ounce, skinless, boneless, drained)
Extra virgin olive oil	1 tablespoon
Fresh lemon juice	2 tablespoons
Red onion	¼ cup (minced)
Pepper	¼ teaspoon (freshly ground)
Cream cheese	4 tablespoons (can use reduced fat)
Pumpernickel bread	8 slices
Tomatoes	8 slices

Romaine lettuce	2 leaves (large, cut in half)

Method:

Combine the oil, pepper, onion, lemon juice and the salmon in a medium sized bowl. Take the bread slices and apply cream cheese to them. Layer at least ½ cup of the salmon salad on top of the cream cheese. Top off with 2 tomatoes and a piece of romaine lettuce and close the sandwich to grill it.

If you have a Panini maker, cook on it until you see the cheese starting to melt and the bread turning brown.

If you don't have a Panini maker, take a grilling pan or a skillet and coat it well with cooking spray. Let it come up to medium heat then place the Panini inside it. Take a smaller saucepan and place it on top of the Panini to compress it.

Make sure to weigh the smaller saucepan down to really compress the sandwich. Cook for 3-4minutes and then remove weight and cook the other side for 2-3 minutes, using the same technique.

Serve:

Serve hot or cold with your favorite beverage.

Salmon BLT Panini
Nutritional Value per Serving:

Calories: 352

Carbohydrates: 48.8g

Cholesterol: 25mg

Fat: 10.9g

Saturated Fat: 6g

Sodium: 741mg

Protein: 16.8g

Fiber: 3.7g

Serving Size: 4

Preparation Time: 10minutes

Cooking Time: 20minutes

Ingredients:

Mayonnaise	¼ cup
Lemon zest	1 teaspoon
Fresh lemon juice	1 teaspoon
Fresh dill leaves	2 tablespoons
Multigrain bread	8 slices (½ inch thick)
Smoked salmon	6 ounces
Arugula	1 cup (divided)
Tomatoes	3 (medium, sliced)

Method:

Take a medium sized bowl and combine the lemon zest, lemon juice, the dill and the mayonnaise. Whisk well until they're all combined. Spread some lemon mayonnaise on 1 side each of the slice. Layer some smoked salmon and arugula on top of it. Now add two slices of tomato before closing the sandwich.

If you have a Panini maker, cook on it until you see the bread turning brown. If you don't have a Panini maker, take a grilling pan or a skillet and coat it well with cooking spray. Let it come up to medium heat then place the Panini inside it. Take a smaller saucepan and place it on top of the Panini to compress it.

Make sure to weigh the smaller saucepan down to really compress the sandwich. Cook for 3-4minutes and then remove weight and cook the other side for 2-3 minutes, using the same technique.

Serve:

Serve hot or cold with your favorite beverage.

Green Goddess Grilled Cheese Panini

Nutritional Value per Serving:

Calories: 130

Carbohydrates: 2.0g

Cholesterol: 5mg

Fat: 13g

Saturated Fat: 2.5g

Sodium: 260mg

Protein: 0.0g

Fiber: 3.7g

Serving Size: 4-6

Preparation Time: 15 minutes

Cooking Time: 15 minutes

Ingredients:

Garlic clove	1 (finely chopped)
Anchovy	1 (oil packed, finely chopped)
Lime zest	1 teaspoon

Fresh Italian parsley	3 tablespoons (chopped)
Fresh tarragon	2 tablespoons (chopped)
Fresh cilantro	2 tablespoons (chopped)
Fresh basil	1 tablespoon (chopped)
Shallot	1 tablespoon (finely chopped)
Djon mustard	¼ teaspoon
Cream cheese	2 ounces (cut in smaller pieces)
Mozzarella	1 cup (shredded)
Sharp cheddar	1 cup (shredded)
Sour dough bread	8-12 slices
Extra virgin olive oil	2 tablespoons

Method:

Use a food processor to pulse the anchovies and garlic together until they form a thick paste. Add in the tarragon, cilantro, shallot, mustard, parsley, lime zest and cream cheese and pulse again to blend all the ingredients together. Take the mixture out in a medium sized bowl and stir the cheddar and mozzarella cheese into the mixture.

Spoon a generous helping of the cheese mixture on to a slice of bread. Close the sandwich with the other slice and brush some olive oil on both sides before grilling it.

If you have a Panini maker, cook on it until you see the bread turning brown. If you don't have a Panini maker, take a grilling pan or a skillet and coat it well with cooking spray. Let it come up to medium heat then place the Panini inside it. Take a smaller saucepan and place it on top of the Panini to compress it.

Make sure to weigh the smaller saucepan down to really compress the sandwich. Cook for 3-4minutes and then remove weight and cook the other side for 2-3 minutes, using the same technique.

Serve:

Serve hot or cold with your favorite beverage.

Tomato, Feta and Oregano Panini

Nutritional Value per Serving:

Calories: 239

Carbohydrates: 0.0g

Cholesterol: 0.0mg

Fat: 27.0g

Saturated Fat: 4.0g

Sodium: 1.0mg

Protein: 0.0g

Fiber: 0.0g

Serving Size: 1

Preparation Time: 5 minutes

Cooking Time: 5 minutes

Ingredients:

Olive bread	2 slices
Olive oil	2 tablespoons
Greek feta cheese	1 ounce

Tomato	2 (sliced, seeds removed)
Fresh oregano leaves	1 bunch
Salt and Pepper	According to taste

Method:

Brush the olive bread well with the olive oil. Layer the bottom slice completely with feta cheese then top off with the tomato slices. Season the tomatoes with salt, pepper and some olive oil before adding the oregano leaves before closing the sandwich.

If you have a Panini maker, cook on it until you see the bread turning brown. If you don't have a Panini maker, take a grilling pan or a skillet and coat it well with cooking spray. Let it come up to medium heat then place the Panini inside it. Take a smaller saucepan and place it on top of the Panini to compress it.

Make sure to weigh the smaller saucepan down to really compress the sandwich. Cook for 3-4minutes and then remove weight and cook the other side for 2-3 minutes, using the same technique.

Serve:

Serve hot or cold with your favorite beverage.

Eggplant Panini with Pesto
Nutritional Value per Serving:

Calories: 336

Carbohydrates: 50g

Cholesterol: 0mg

Fat: 8.5g

Saturated Fat: 2.5g

Sodium: 394mg

Protein: 11.4g

Fiber: 3.8g

Serving Size: 4

Preparation Time: 15 minutes

Cooking Time: 15 minutes

Ingredients:

Olive oil	3 tablespoons
Egg plant	1 (large, sliced)
French bread	12 oz (cut into 4 pieces and sliced in half)
Mozzarella cheese	4 slices
Tomato	8 slices (thinly sliced)
Basil pesto	2 tablespoons

Method:

Season the egg plants with some salt and set aside for 30 minutes. Sprinkle the olive oil over the eggplants and season some more with salt and pepper. Cook on a grill for 7-8 minutes or until they start to soften, making sure to turn them while cooking.

Layer the bread with 3 pieces of grilled eggplant, ½ a tablespoon of basil pesto, 1 slice of mozzarella and 2 slices of tomato each. Close the sandwich and brush with olive oil before grilling.

Spoon a generous helping of the cheese mixture on to a slice of bread. Close the sandwich with the other slice and brush some olive oil on both sides before grilling it.

If you have a Panini maker, cook on it until you see the bread turning brown. If you don't have a Panini maker, take a grilling pan or a skillet and coat it well with cooking spray.

Let it come up to medium heat then place the Panini inside it. Take a smaller saucepan and place it on top of the Panini to compress it.

Make sure to weigh the smaller saucepan down to really compress the sandwich. Cook for 3-4minutes and then remove weight and cook the other side for 2-3 minutes, using the same technique.

Serve:

Serve hot or cold with your favorite beverage.

Simple Salami Panini

Nutritional Value per Serving:

Calories: 397

Carbohydrates: 22g

Cholesterol: 71mg

Fat: 26g

Saturated Fat: 13g

Sodium: 1074mg

Protein: 18g

Fiber: 1g

Serving Size: 4

Preparation Time: 10 minutes

Cooking Time: 15 minutes

Ingredients:

Salami	4 ounces (sliced thinly)
Fontina cheese	4 ounces (sliced thinly)

Pepperoncini	4 (jarred, sliced thinly, lengthwise)
Olive oil	2 tablespoons
Sour dough bread	8 slices

Method:

Layer the bread with some salami, the pepperoncini and the Fontina cheese as well. Close the sandwich and brush with olive oil before grilling the sandwich.

Spoon a generous helping of the cheese mixture on to a slice of bread. Close the sandwich with the other slice and brush some olive oil on both sides before grilling it.

If you have a Panini maker, cook on it until you see the bread turning brown. If you don't have a Panini maker, take a grilling pan or a skillet and coat it well with cooking spray. Let it come up to medium heat then place the Panini inside it. Take a smaller saucepan and place it on top of the Panini to compress it.

Make sure to weigh the smaller saucepan down to really compress the sandwich. Cook for 3-4minutes and then remove weight and cook the other side for 2-3 minutes, using the same technique.

Serve:

Serve hot or cold with your favorite beverage.

Horse radish, Roast beef and Cheddar Panini

Nutritional Value per Serving:

Calories: 524

Carbohydrates: 43g

Cholesterol: 92mg

Fat: 27g

Saturated Fat: 14g

Sodium: 1070mg

Protein: 28g

Fiber: 4g

Serving Size: 4

Preparation Time: 15 minutes

Cooking Time: 15 minutes

Ingredients:

Cream cheese	4 ounces (softened)
Horse radish	2 tablespoons (prepared)
Sourdough bread	8 slices
Romaine lettuce	1 head (remove tough ribs)
Deli roast beef	8 ounces (thinly sliced)
Cheddar	4 ounces (sliced)
Olive oil	2 tablespoons

Method:

Tale a small bowl and combine the horse radish and the cream cheese. Spread this mixture on 4 slices. Add a layer of lettuce, roast beef and cheddar. Close the sandwich and brush with olive oil before grilling it.

If you have a Panini maker, cook on it until you see the bread turning brown. If you don't have a Panini maker, take a grilling pan or a skillet and coat it well with cooking spray. Let it come up to medium heat then place the Panini inside it. Take a smaller saucepan and place it on top of the Panini to compress it.

Make sure to weigh the smaller saucepan down to really compress the sandwich. Cook for 3-4minutes and then remove weight and cook the other side for 2-3 minutes, using the same technique.

Serve:

Serve hot or cold with your favorite beverage.

www.ingramcontent.com/pod-product-compliance
Lightning Source LLC
Chambersburg PA
CBHW080420290526
45791CB00008BA/2352